MW00906072

The Lazy Woman's Guide to Yoga

The Lazy Woman's Guide to Yoga

Taylore Daniel

Text Copyright 2017 © Taylore Daniel

Illustrations Copyright 2017 © Taylore Daniel

ISBN- 978-0-9735662-3-9 (electronic book)

ISBN – 978-0-9735662-8-4 (softcover book)

www.tayloredaniel.com

No part of this book may be reproduced, utilized or transmitted in any form or by any means, electronic or mechanical–including photocopying, recording on any information storage or retrieval system–without written permission from the publisher, except for brief quotations or inclusion in a review. All rights reserved.

Cover Design by Taylore Daniel

Cover Image by Dreamstime

DISCLAIMER: Neither the publisher nor the authors are engaged in rendering professional advice or services to the individual reader. The ideas, procedures, and suggestions contained in this e-book are not intended as a substitute for consulting with a physician. All matters regarding health require medical supervision. Neither the author nor the publisher shall be liable or responsible for any loss or damage allegedly arising from any information or suggestions in this book.

Contents

Dedication

With thanks to all yoga teachers,

and all yoga students,

in all traditions.

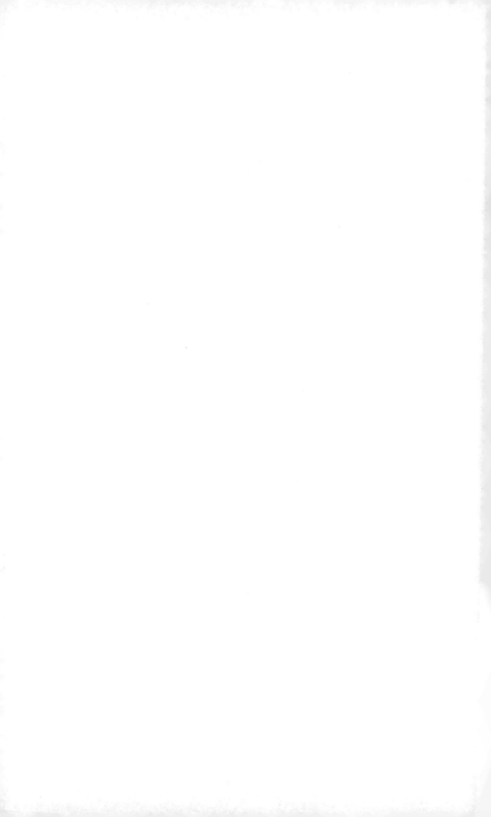

Introduction

According to recent studies, "Sitting is the new smoking." And it's largely because of our high-tech world with its cornucopia of online activities.

Whether its YouTube, Netflix, Facebook, email, texting, blogging, Twittering or work, a lot of our day is spent sitting in front of screens.

Basically, the amount of downtime spent sitting is going up.

And this lack of activity is playing havoc with our health. Our human body is like a pool of water. It needs movement to get the blood and oxygen circulating. Without this, our systems become stagnant. And that leads to trouble.

So what is a solution?

Yoga is one superb way to keep ourselves moving. And there's nothing better than being in the energy of a roomful of like-minded people who share a love of yoga. Except that getting our yoga gear together, driving to the yoga studio, taking a class, chatting after, then showering and changing for our next activity can feel like a real time bite.

And if we're driving through traffic to get to and from our class, we may end up more stressed than relaxed by our efforts.

Even if we have a nearby yoga studio and regular classes, we may crave more than one hour of physical activity a day to break up our screen-filled lives. Yet we may feel unsure about how to incorporate this into our daily stream of errands.

My aim with this guide is to help you easily and effortlessly add more yoga into your life, wherever you're at — time-wise, health-wise, location-wise, motivation-wise or otherwise.

I hope *The Lazy Woman's Guide to Yoga* inspires you to do more yoga by making it so luxuriously easy, that it feels downright lazy.

First Things First

Is it possible to do yoga without a mat?

Absolutely! One of the core tenets of *The Lazy Woman's Guide to Yoga* is that it can be done at the same time you carry on with your daily leisure and work activities. No need to get down on the floor. No need to carry around any special equipment in the form of mats, blocks, bands or blankets.

Can I do it without special yoga wear?

Yes! No special clothing is required. This is another incredible benefit of *The Lazy Woman's Guide to Yoga*. The whole premise of this guide is that you can do yoga anywhere. That means you can wear anything from a sundress to a business suit, from flip-flops to high heels.

Can I really do yoga while I'm just sitting on my sofa? Or shopping for cereal? Or surfing the net?

Yes, you can! In fact you can do it lounging by the pool, visiting your neighbors, scanning tabloids in the supermarket, waiting for your accountant's appointment, sitting on a flight, working in an office, riding an elevator, or any single other place you choose.

You'll be given a simple and effortless way to integrate yoga movements and poses into every single activity, or inactivity, of your life so you can choose what works for where you are, who you're with, and how you feel at any given moment. You can break out a move in your office, in your car, on your sofa, walking, in front of your laptop … even with one hand on the mouse!

How will I remember all the moves and poses when I'm alone and without a teacher?

This is one of the highlights of *The Lazy Woman's Guide to Yoga*.

Using a simple acronym, you'll easily remember a group of yoga moves done in a specific order. And you'll only ever have to remember one word to trigger either an entire yoga set, or a single yoga move that fits whatever situation you're in.

Each part of this system comes with variations that range in subtlety and level of challenge. But all you'll need to do is remember one single word. Everything will flow from that.

Do I have to breathe in any funny ways?

Breath is one of the greatest ways to add "oomph" to a movement.

Breath can make a move more effortless by powering up the body, giving it more energy. And at the same time, breath can make a move more challenging, because powering up a move increases the energy you expend.

The only conscious breathing I'm going to mention in this book, however, has to do with a) deepening and slowing the breath or b) synchronizing it with a movement. Both have incredible benefits, which include:

- changing our moods and emotions
- improving our respiratory system
- strengthening our nervous system
- improving blood and oxygen circulation
- massaging the internal organs
- regulating hormones
- balancing the digestive system

What are some other benefits of yoga, in general?

In addition to the benefits listed above, yoga:

- develops muscle
- increases physical strength
- increases tendon and ligament resilience
- strengthens joints
- enhances pain management
- increases flexibility
- adds bone mass
- increases energy and vitality
- improves balance and coordination
- regulates blood pressure
- increases oxygen and blood circulation to the brain, improving clarity, attention and memory
- strengthens the heart
- brings a greater sense of relaxation
- and offers profound stress relief

Considering that stress is thought to be the number one cause of disease, this one benefit alone is worth the minimal effort and bountiful joy of practicing yoga. And it's my goal to make this practice so effortless and convenient, that you'll want to fill your life with stolen moments of yoga with the same delicious anticipation of a stolen kiss from your lover.

What is the 70% rule?

Above all else, remember this:

Never give more than 70% of your effort to any single stretch.

When it comes to stretching, giving 100% can do more harm than good. If you've met people who have injured themselves during yoga or other stretching activities, you may hear them say they wanted "to give it all they got." This is a part of our cultural conditioning, this drive to give 100% to everything.

When it comes to positions that involve endurance, like holding your arms out, yes, 100% is great. But stretching is different than endurance. If you want to see how long you can hold your arms out, assuming there is absolutely no joint pain in doing so, you're building muscle. But the stretching part of a movement should feel entirely effortless. Only the endurance part should feel challenging.

You may think that you won't see any progress in your flexibility if you don't give 100% to your stretches. But quite the opposite is true, because the body has a built-in protection system when it comes to stretching.

When it feels it is nearing capacity, it contracts as a way of protecting the tendons, ligaments, and muscle fibers. Thus, if we are striving against this protective response by giving

100%, we're pushing while our body is pulling. And this, very simply, can lead to injuries.

Conversely, if we give just 70% to any stretching movement, our body stays relaxed. And it's in relaxing that our flexibility naturally increases. So that what takes 70% of our effort today, only takes 60% tomorrow. We can then increase our range of movement by 10% to bring it back up to 70%… and so on.

Which is to say, by only stretching to 70% capacity, we are increasing our endurance, our strength and our flexibility. But we are doing it in a way that is safe.

This is the easier, more effortless and enjoyable way, some might even say the "lazy way" to practice yoga.

Okay. So what do I do first?

The heart of *The Lazy Woman's Guide to Yoga* is to have a method to practice yoga that fits into your life, easily and effortlessly, in every single way.

This includes having a mental system whereby as soon as you think of doing yoga, you'll have a whole orderly repertoire of moves that will come to mind.

Basically, this system is so easy that you'll just have to think of one word, "First", and you'll have an entire yoga set at the ready, one that is easy to use anywhere, anytime—no mats, floor work, or special attire needed.

So why are you going to think of the word "First"?

Because "F.I.R.S.T." is being used as an acronym, with each letter representing a word, and with each word representing a yoga move and a few of its variations.

Soon, as you are waking up, waiting in a line, sitting at your laptop, or lounging by the seaside, you'll think "FIRST."

And you'll mentally scroll through the yoga options from the fabulous FIRST menu, until you come to one that feels just right for the occasion.

By the end of this guide you'll have at the tip of your fingers, at the forefront of your mind, a tool to practice yoga wherever you find yourself.

A brief overview of F.I.R.S.T. :

"F" is for FLYING (yes, you heard that right, flying, like a bird)

"I" is for INFINITY (symbolized since ancient times by what looks like a horizontal figure-8: ∞)

"R" is for ROCK (imagine the way rocks can be stacked one atop another in perfect balance, the same way the bones of our body are when we're in perfect balance and alignment)

"S" is for SPIRAL (winding in curves)

"T" is for TAPPING (think acupressure points)

How long / how many repetitions should I do of each movement?

All moves can be done in whatever way best fits your time and motivations. If you want to fill in a couple of free minutes before an appointment or while waiting for a traffic light, you can choose one move and repeat it. Simply scroll through the letters of F.I.R.S.T., from "F" to "T" and choose the most appealing, or appropriate, move for the occasion.

If you want to put structured mini-breaks into your screen time, there are a few options. For instance, doing eight repetitions, or perhaps three minutes, from each movement category is one way. Or simply choosing a time-period like five or fifteen minutes and filling it with a rotating, ordered series of movements from the F.I.R.S.T. menu is another option. In the last chapter, I've included more detail.

Now let's begin.

FLYING

INFINITY

ROCK

SPIRAL

TAPPING

3

Flying

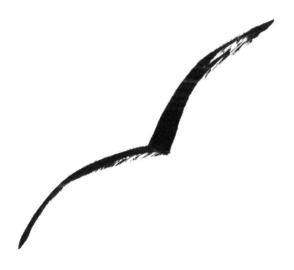

TAYLORE DANIEL

*

F. I. R. S. T.

F IS FOR FLYING

Flying is an amazing, fun, effortless movement with profound benefits.

If you only used this one single movement in all its infinite glory, you'd experience a transformation.

Your stress levels would fall. Tension in your shoulders would lessen. Your arm muscles and back muscles would get stronger and suppler. Your energy would increase. Not to mention that once you get into the flow of it, flying feels absolutely wonderful.

And it has variations that work for every circumstance. For instance, subtle variations can be practiced while standing in line at the bank or at a café reading the newspaper. Expansive variations can be done wherever you have the space and freedom, from your living room to the park.

At the simplest level, your arms begin by your sides and you raise them up above your head. But to bring a whole new dimension of ease to this movement, imagine your arms are like wings, floating effortlessly through the air without gravity, as though lifted by the wind.

If you close your eyes and envision your arms as broad and powerful as the wings of a pelican, crane, or falcon, you'll also notice a more expansive and graceful range of motion.

Try it and see. I'd love to hear what you think.

TIP: Another mental image that can be used while flying is… swimming.

When standing in the water with your arms at your sides, it doesn't take long for them to effortlessly float upwards. The buoyancy of the water lifts them. Likewise, using this image will lift your arms with an unexpected lightness.

Is there a way to make this move more challenging?

Yes there is. Speed.

But there is a paradox here, as it is slowness that makes this move more challenging. The slower you go, the more you'll feel like you're lifting weights, and the faster your muscles will grow.

In fact, studies show that when it comes to building strength, the important thing is not to lift a lot of weight, but to lift until we reach failure—until we can't do one more repetition.

This is great news on so many levels.

For one, it means we don't have to lift weights to build strength. And why is this good?

Because it means we can build our strength anywhere, anytime, without the need for accessories.

After all, you can't exactly lug around weights in your purse in the off chance you have a moment to squeeze in some strength-building exercises. But you can fly ever so slowly nearly anywhere, and at anytime. No equipment needed.

So let's get started.

*

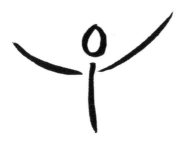

FLYING – PELICAN

Begin with your arms out at your sides, parallel to the floor. Then raise and lower them. The range can be just a few inches if you're out in public. Or above your head if you have the space and the right environment. Keep your shoulders relaxed.

OPTION: Synchronize your movements with your breath, inhaling as your arms rise, exhaling as they fall. Deep breathing creates mental clarity, releases emotional stress, and carries more oxygen to the cells, which raises energy and creates health.

OPTION: Have your palms facing up. Or facing down. Play with both these styles, and feel the dramatically different stretch in your arms and forearms.

*

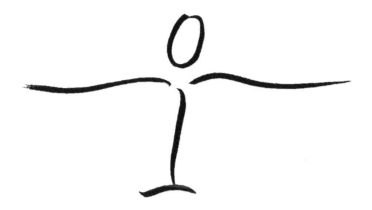

FLYING – GLIDING

Birds with large wingspans glide elegantly through the sky, their wings making tiny adjustments and corrections to deal with airflow patterns.

In this gliding pose, put your arms out to the sides horizontally (parallel to the ground) and hold. This is even more challenging than raising and lowering your arms slowly. It won't take long to feel the burn of your muscles firing up.

OPTION: Glide with your arms held up in a V shape.

OPTION: When in public, glide with your arms down and closer to your sides, like an inverted V. While this might seem too easy to be useful, holding this pose for any length of time will activate a number of arm muscles. Gravity works just as well as a resistance band.

OPTION: Move your arms up and down within a two or three inch range anywhere within the flying spectrum.

This is a surprisingly challenging variation, as it is easier to swing our arms up and down fully than to move them within a small range, especially if it involves hovering them around the horizontal line. If your range of motion is limited, this will be a perfect fit.

OPTION: Keep your hands and wrists rigid as your arms move up and down. Or aim to capture the grace of a ballerina, whose arms flow like the branches of a willow tree. Experiment.

NOTE: If you feel any discomfort or pinching sensations, reduce the range of motion and keep the range closer to your body (instead of on a horizontal line). Also, slow the movement down so you can control it. Another option is to simply visualize and imagine yourself doing the movement. Wherever thoughts go, energy flows.

*

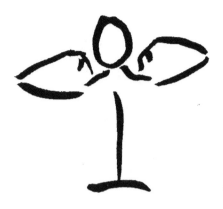

FLYING – HUMMINGBIRD

You might enjoy having a smaller wingspan, which involves crooking your elbow so your hands rest on your shoulders while moving your arms up and down. This is a handy variation to use in a tight space.

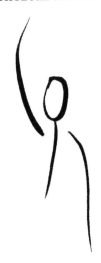

FLYING – ONE-WINGED FLIGHT

This is the perfect move when you've got your Smartphone, TV remote, or computer mouse in hand. In fact, one of my arms is flying as I edit this.

Simply raise and lower one arm at a time, changing your mouse, converter or cellphone to the other hand when you tire, and flying with the other arm. This is a great way to get in some yoga while enjoying your leisure time or screen time.

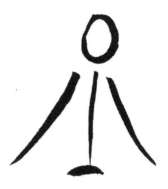

FLYING – BREATH

One powerful yet relaxing way to fly is to power your arms entirely with your breath.

Begin with your arms loose and relaxed at your sides. Inhale deeply into your chest, so your ribs expand and physically move your arms as you inhale. Imagine that with each inhale, your arms begin to fill with air like balloons, gently lifting away from your body, then returning to your sides on the exhale.

Now imagine that each inhalation adds a bit more helium to your limbs, allowing them to float slightly higher each time. Flying that is powered by the breath is a distinct experience. It is very calming. Very relaxing.

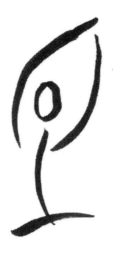

FLYING – AT AN ANGLE

With this fun flying variation, lean from the waist to one side as you raise your arms up. Bring your body back to the center as you lower your arms down. Then repeat on the opposite side.

This is a remarkably good stretch for the rib cage and creates suppleness in the spine, which increases spinal fluid to all the joints of the body. And supple joints are youthful joints.

4

Infinity

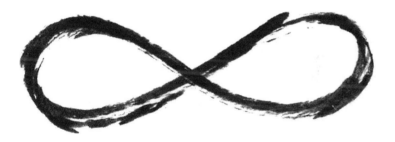

*

TAYLORE DANIEL

*

F. I. R. S. T.
I IS FOR INFINITY YOGA

Like flying, this one series of movements would be enough to carry you through the end of your days.

And it's fitting that this move is called "Infinity," as there are infinite variations. Everything from the most subtle—almost invisible—movements to the most expansive and wildest full-body versions.

This coterie of infinity movements can work as a go-to when you're someplace where, for the life of you, you cannot imagine how to fit in some yoga. There will be a move you can depend upon at any time, anywhere within this chapter, whether it's shopping at the mall, brushing your teeth, browsing through a book store, texting, watching a movie, surfing the net, or tanning on the beach.

This chapter is, in fact, part of a full system I've developed called the Infinity Yoga Method©. In my upcoming book of the same name, I'll explain it in further detail, including its background, benefits, and many more complex and challenging variations for those who really want to get their heart rate up.

The moves themselves are easy snippets of fun that, like all the moves and poses in *The Lazy Woman's Guide to Yoga*, are completely effortless. They can be practiced right in the midst of our laziest, most halcyon moments of do-nothing bliss.

Or... they can be an antidote to our preponderance of time spent on tablets, smartphones, laptops, and home computers.

With this in mind, the first few variations in this series of infinity moves addresses the areas of our bodies most affected by the repetitive and locked-in positions of abundant screen time.

And these mini-breaks are especially terrific, because we don't even have to leave our post in front of the screen to increase our health and relieve physical stress.

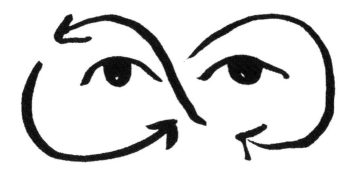

INFINITY YOGA – EYES

Let's begin with the eyes.

When we're gazing at a screen, as so many of us are doing not only during our leisure time but at work as well, the muscles behind our eyes become locked into a certain position.

This is related to how close or far away the screen is from our face. And it also has to do with how long we lock on without using our peripheral or distance vision.

By taking even 30 seconds here and there to do some eye exercises, we're stretching our eye muscles and giving them a little workout, increasing their strength and suppleness.

If we don't do this, our eyes eventually lose their capacity to jump easily between objects near and far. They become less flexible. And before we know it, they become so locked into seeing near that seeing far requires glasses.

We aren't likely to give up our tablets, smartphones, laptops and t.v.'s, so let's make sure we keep all our necessary body parts in tip-top shape to enjoy them.

In this first infinity eye exercise, simply imagine a sideways figure eight (the infinity symbol) in front of your face and let your eyes follow it.

Begin with your eyes to the right, drop them down, then come in towards the nose. You'll be cross-eyed for a millisecond as your eyes pass over the nose bridge and rise up and to the left. Then swoop your eyes in a downwards arc back in towards the center again. Repeat.

After a time, change direction.

*

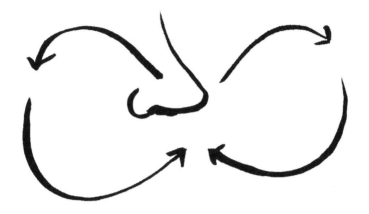

INFINITY YOGA –

NECK AND NECK BY A NOSE!

In this infinity move, we're not actually exercising our nose. But we'll focus on our nose in order to exercise... our neck.

Yes, it's true. Strange but effective.

Essentially, we gently move the tip of our nose in the pattern of the infinity symbol.

Imagine your nose is a marker and you are softly drawing the infinity symbol onto a whiteboard. You'll notice that indeed, all the small muscles of your neck are getting a lovely little stretch.

You can also draw a vertical infinity symbol (the figure eight) against an imaginary whiteboard to work another set of small neck muscles.

The eyes and the neck are the first delicate muscles to pay the price when we lock on a screen for long periods of time. These two small eye and nose movements alone can really make a difference in bringing health and wellness.

Upcoming moves also relax the neck muscles, but include the shoulders and other parts of the body as well, whereas the nose movement targets the neck specifically.

*

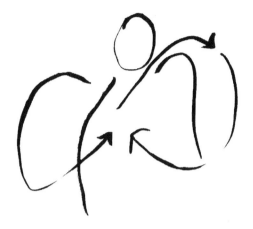

INFINITY YOGA – SHOULDERS

Begin moving one shoulder up towards your ear, then in a circle that reaches out sideways. Drop the shoulder down and circle it up and back to the heart line, which I'll also call the center point.

As our shoulder comes back to center, the opposite shoulder takes up the movement, as though in a relay. This shoulder now circles up, then out sideways away from the center line in the opposite direction. Then downwards and back towards the heart, where the other shoulder takes up the movement again.

While moving your shoulders, allow your arms to fall loosely at your sides, the trunk of your body swaying gently as it follows the movement of your shoulders, your rib cage getting a nice stretch along the way.

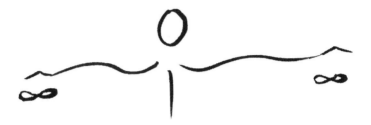

INFINITY YOGA – WRISTS

Wrists are taken for granted in the grand scheme of things. But there's a lot of stress put on wrists. And for anyone who's had a repetitive strain injury and been unable to use their wrists fully, there's an immediate awareness of just how much is expected of this small joint.

Not to mention that in our techie society, our wrists perform a lot of tight, repetitive, small movements, which demand some relief.

The infinity moves for the wrists are to be performed with the 70% rule. This means giving only 70% of your effort to any stretch. We do not want to cause a counter-pull, because it's just plain counter-productive.

Gently and slowly are the key words here. Not to mention that the slower you go, the more luxurious the sensation.

To begin, put your arms out to your side (parallel to the

ground) with your shoulders and arms relaxed. Move your hands in gentle infinity shapes, as though the tips of your fingers are drawing the symbol on screens to either side of you.

The palms face down for one half of the infinity sign, then turn up for the second half of the infinity sign. This brings circulation and increased flexibility to your wrists, provides a lovely stretch to the forearms, and builds muscle in your upper arms.

*

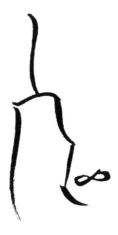

INFINITY YOGA – ANKLES

This one is great because it can be done unobtrusively while sitting almost anywhere: under the table at a café or restaurant, at your desk, lounging by the seaside, in the bath... The list goes on.

The benefit is supple ankles. Later, we will learn moves to increase ankle strength, and together these contribute to balance. Balance is important stuff, especially when hiking, climbing, or dealing with slippery or cracked sidewalks.

The movement itself involves turning one ankle at a time (or both if you like) in smooth infinity patterns. The trick is to make the movement as graceful as possible, and to work out the jerky, awkward bits. It is a small but interesting challenge to aim for grace in every single movement.

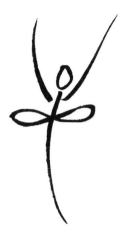

INFINITY YOGA – RIB CAGE

With the arms up (or down), let your rib cage guide this movement. Imagine your rib cage as a round ball that you are guiding in an infinity movement through space, bringing the whole trunk of your body along for the ride.

This can be done sitting or standing.

Benefits include an expanded rib cage, which means greater lung capacity. As well, it brings circulation and relaxation to the back muscles.

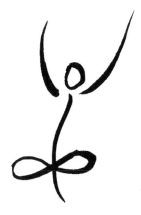

INFINITY YOGA – HIPS

Done from a standing position, arms up or down, you draw the infinity symbol with your hips as though on a level plane.

You're not aiming for the symbol to look like it is drawn here, with ups and downs, but rather with your hips doing backward and forward movements as you trace the curves into the air.

Sitting is the new smoking, and this movement is a direct response to the problem.

It brings circulation to the hip joints, opening and balancing them when they have become tight with too much sitting.

Tip: Keep your knees softly bent.

*

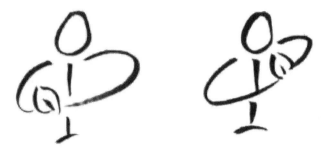

INFINITY YOGA – UPPER BODY

This fun movement starts by putting your hands together in prayer pose at chest level. Aim your hands first in one direction with palms together, then swoop them in the opposite direction as though tracing the infinity symbol through the air with the tips of your fingers.

This is a superb exercise for all the joints in the upper body, from the shoulders to the elbows to the wrists. The rib cage, upper back and chest also get a wonderful stretch.

OPTION: Instead of tracing the infinity symbol at chest level, trace it at head level or even above your head. Always aim for a smooth, flowing rhythm.

*

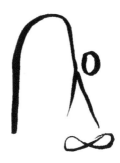

INFINITY YOGA – DRAWING ON THE FLOOR

This is a surprisingly effective stretch that you'll feel along the outside of your hips and legs, as well as through the waist and rib cage.

From a standing position, begin by bending over and letting your arms fall. If you have issues with eye pressure or blood pressure, skip this pose or modify it by keeping your head up and facing a wall.

With your hands tracing the infinity symbol on the ground, allow the entire trunk of your body to follow along. The infinity sign can extend far to each side and even sway over and behind your ankles if that's comfortable.

The closer your feet are to each other, the more you'll feel the stretch in your hips. The farther apart they are, the more you'll feel the stretch in your waist.

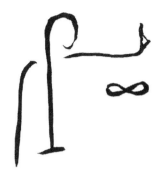

INFINITY YOGA – ARM TO SIDE

This is one of my favorite movements, as it is intense, yet subtle. It creates a delicious stretch all the way through the elbow and forearm to the tip of the forefinger.

It can be done sitting or standing, facing forward or to the side, as in the illustration above.

The benefit to keeping both eyes focused on the fingernail of your raised forefinger is that your neck gets a welcome stretch. And keeping the head turned to the side intensifies the stretch along your arm—so much so that your finger will tingle. It also exercises your eyes.

Begin by raising your arm out to the side, keeping you elbow and wrist still.

Bend your hand at a 90-degree angle to your wrist (or

TAYLORE DANIEL

according to your ability). If you need to, bend your elbow
until the forefinger of your hand points directly up.

With your forefinger pointing up, your thumb covers the tips
of your middle, ring and pinkie fingers. This leaves a hole in
the center, as in the illustration.

Now imagine tracing the infinity symbol with the pad of
your forefinger, as though on a wall to your side. While you
will notice only the fingertip tracing infinity into the air,
the movement itself originates from the shoulder joint. The
elbow and wrist are locked into position.

This is a great mini-break movement while on the computer,
facing forward with one hand on the mouse. Try it and see.

OPTION: Put both arms out to the side holding this hand
position. It's a terrific stretch while you are occupied reading
or watching a screen.

5

Rock

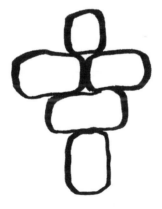

*

47

TAYLORE DANIEL

*

48

F. I. R. S. T.

R IS FOR ROCK

Anytime you're waiting in line, or for the laundry to finish, or the water to boil …

Anytime you're perusing cereal options in the grocery store, magazines in the shop, or clothing at a local boutique…

Anytime you're ambling from the living room to the bedroom, the office to the cooler, or the kitchen to the front door… you have the opportunity to get in a little yoga.

The "rock" pose I describe here isn't the traditional yogic sitting-on-your-heels pose. Because obviously, the above situations would not be ideal places to hunker down onto the floor and sit on our feet.

The majority of these rock poses involve solid standing poses… balancing on one foot.

Sound too simple?

To maintain balance while standing on one foot, our body must make a thousand little adjustments and corrections every second, and each of these involves a muscle firing off and getting into the action. The biggest benefit of all is that the ankle-foot complex is strengthened, meaning that we have increased control of our balance. This means fewer lower limb injuries, increased agility and sports performance, and better fall prevention. As well, these poses develop our large leg muscles, increasing our metabolism.

Another great thing is that you can do this movement in public without being noticed… unless you tip over, of course.

Safety

This brings us to the issue of safety. Only do this movement when it is safe. If your balance isn't a sure thing, don't stand next to an open fire or cliff edge. Or without something or someone nearby to grab onto.

In fact, an option is to keep the toe of your non-weight bearing foot touching the ground so you have a safety net. Alternately, practice close to the edge of a table or chair that you can latch onto if need be.

Now that I've given you the caveats, let's take a look at some variations on this most basic, but challenging, move. It's become one of my personal favorites, and it gives me a huge sense of satisfaction to forever be finding more difficult one-legged positions.

*

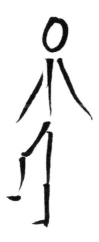

ROCK – Balance 1

We'll start with the most basic move, so you can test out your balance. Simply lift one foot off the floor and see how long you can comfortably hold this. For an added challenge, rise up onto tip toe.

*

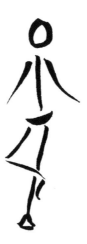

ROCK – BALANCE 2

If you find that relaxing, tuck your lifted foot behind your ankle or perch it against your shin, thereby removing the safety net of having your lifted foot close to the ground. Hold as long as you can or until the line-up at the grocery store, bank or airport check-in moves.

*

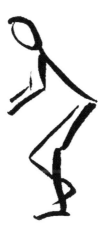

ROCK – LEANING OVER

With one foot off the ground, bend at the hips and try to remain balanced on one foot as you adjust your height.

This could be used if, for example, you're in the grocery story or bookshop and want to eyeball items at different levels, some on low shelves and some on high shelves... all the while continuing to stand on just one leg.

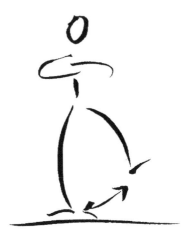

ROCK – PENDULUM

This one can be done waiting in line-ups too. It takes your attention off the frustration of waiting and on to the fabulous boost you get by improving your balance, coordination and large muscle groups all at once.

The movement is not the focus in this pose. The focus is on how still and balanced you can keep your body while moving just one limb. Start by lifting one leg straight out to the side in a swinging motion, sweeping it out to the side and back. Keep the trunk of your body aligned. Your arms will hang loose by your side, unless you need to flail them about a bit to keep your balance.

*

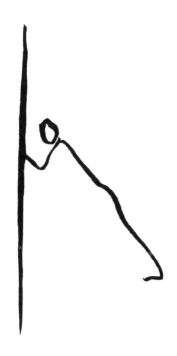

ROCK – WALL PLANK

The Lazy Woman's Guide to Yoga doesn't involve getting down on the floor for this plank. Instead, simply brace your hands against a wall, hold your stomach tight and tuck in your bottom. With your heels down, your calves get a great stretch. If this heel stretch feels like more than 70%, lift your heels up.

While this version of the plank, versus the traditional position on the floor, takes longer to reach a point of failure, it ultimately achieves the same results.

And you can work it in as you walk down the hall from your kitchen to your bedroom, achieving a mini-workout... the lazy way.

OPTION: Hold the plank position against the wall using only your fingertips.

OPTION: Do a push-up against the wall for variety.

*

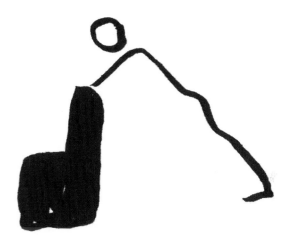

ROCK – SOFA PLANK

Doing a plank against the back or arm of a stable chair or sofa puts less pressure on your shoulder and wrist joints, because you aren't at full horizontal placement. Better still, by not having to get down on the floor, you don't have to worry about the last time you vacuumed the rug.

Nor do you need to pull out a yoga mat.

Yet you'll get the same benefits of building upper body and core strength, while engaging in a phone conversation, radio program, or Youtube clip.

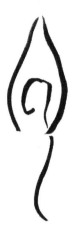

ROCK – REACHING HIGH

So far we've done rock poses standing upright and leaning against something.

This last one has you back on your sofa or chair, or anywhere else for that matter. And the rock aspect is in the position of your arms.

We looked at similar poses in the gliding section of the chapter on Flying. In this specific pose, position your arms directly above your head, hands clasped together. Or for more of a challenge, press your palms flat against each other. Then hold either for a preset period of time, or until your toast pops or your video loads.

The benefits of this simple pose are similar to those you get while Flying, and include a stronger nervous system, increased oxygen to the brain, improved digestion, a shrinking abdominal cavity, increased mental energy and postural corrections.

6

Spiral

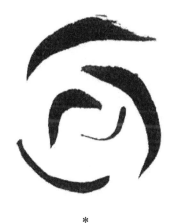

*

TAYLORE DANIEL

*

F. I. R. S. T.

S IS FOR SPIRAL

This is one of the most natural of movements, and you'll find it an absolute delight.

I'll be using the term *spiral* loosely here, because some of the movements are spirals, while other variations are your basic circle.

Anyway... let's get going, as you are going to love this series of movements.

*

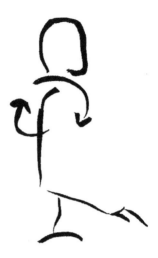

SPIRAL – SHOULDERS CIRCLING UP & DOWN

Move shoulders up, forward, down and around.

You can actually do this movement while both hands are occupied with other activities, like typing on the computer, reading a book or drinking coffee.

After rolling them forward for eight rotations, or whatever time period suits your fancy, reverse direction, rolling your shoulders backwards.

*

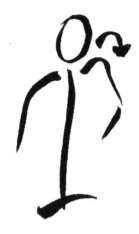

SPIRAL – SHOULDERS CIRCLING SIDE TO SIDE

Instead of rotating your shoulders up and down, roll them out to the side. Then in to the center. This targets different muscles and engages the trunk of the body, activating the muscles of the upper back and chest.

Alternate shoulders with each round and notice your heart rate increase and your breathing deepen. A great energizing move.

*

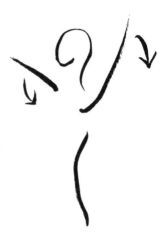

SPIRAL – SHOULDERS DROP FROM ABOVE

Begin with both hands stretched high above your head. As one arm drops forward in front of your body, drop the other arm backwards. And continue to cycle them in opposing directions.

This takes a bit of coordination at first. If you'd like to begin a bit more slowly, instead of bringing your arms completely around in full circles right away, simply let them drop down to the sides of your body and rest. Then repeat.

When this comes easily, instead of resting them at your sides after the drop, keep them moving in big circles until your arms meet again above your head.

Once momentum builds, you'll notice your hips swinging, fueling the movement and making it rhythmic and flowing.

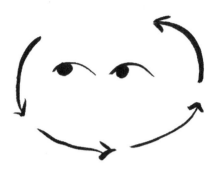

SPIRAL – EYES FOLLOWING THE RIMS

Begin by looking up, then circle your eyes slowly and gently, as though tracing the outline of the rims of your eyes or your environment. First up, then right, down, then left. Rotate in both directions.

The aim is to move them smoothly and slowly, without any skips or stalls. If there is a lot of unevenness, slow down the movement even more. It's an oddly enjoyable challenge to circle the eyes as gracefully as possible.

As with all stretches, only give 70%. You don't want to strain your muscles, and that includes the eyes.

This exercise will increase your peripheral vision, and keep your eye muscles flexible and healthy. It's a great yoga move to do as a screen break.

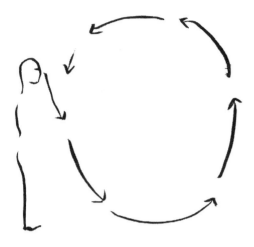

SPIRAL – EYES CIRCLING OUT INTO THE DISTANCE

This spiraling eye movement is particularly important as it exercises the eye muscles responsible for near and far sightedness. And with much of our leisure time being spent in front of screens set close to our faces, our eye muscles can get locked into "close" position, becoming rigid, so that we lose the ability to focus easily into the distance.

In this circular eye motion, instead of shifting our gaze from right to left, or up to down, we're shifting our gaze from near to far.

If you're in a room, this means the far point is the opposite wall or somewhere outside your window. If you're outside, well, the far point is as far as your eye can see. The key point is to move your eyes, not your head, as you follow this circle out, up and back.

Feel free to remove your glasses if it's convenient.

Begin by imagining you are watching a miniature airplane take off from the ground at your feet. It sets off down the runway that is your carpet or perhaps a sidewalk or field.

You imagine this plane taxiing along the ground as far as your eyes can see (e.g., to the edge of your room or the edge of the earth). Then imagine the airplane taking off smoothly into the air, up, up, up, as high as your eyes can follow (indoors, up the wall to the ceiling; outdoors, up into the sky).

Then imagine the airplane flying back towards you in a big arc and gracefully landing back at your feet before continuing down the runway away from you again.

I find this airplane metaphor helpful to keep my eyes tracing this large air-circle smoothly. But use whatever feels best.

*

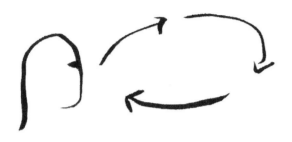

SPIRAL – EYES ON AN EVEN PLANE

I love the sensation of this one, and just can't get enough of it. It can be practiced anywhere, and is a real treat outdoors, though it's just as much fun in a room, an elevator, or looking out a window. As with all the exercises, the aim is to produce a smooth flowing motion.

There's no "up and down" at all in this eye yoga activity. It's all on a level plane. If you're sitting, your eyes will trace everything at sitting level. If you're standing, everything you see will be at standing level.

Very simply, both eyes begin by moving to the right in a wide arc until you're looking off in the distance straight out in front of you. Then your eyes continue their trajectory in a wide arc out to the left, circling back to your nose and off to the right again. This circling movement feels like being on a gently swirling fair ride. Absolutely terrific feeling.

*

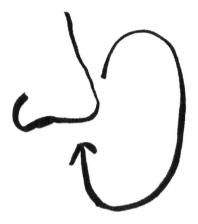

SPIRAL - NOSE

This movement is similar in nature to the earlier infinity movement, in that while we focus on the nose, it is the neck that receives the benefits.

Imagine your nose is a felt pen, and you are drawing a circle on a whiteboard. Repeat eight times in each direction, or as long as it feels good.

It's great for stretching those small neck muscles, which like the eye muscles, can get locked and tense from too much time in one position.

*

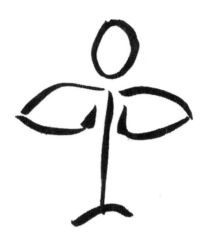

SPIRAL – HAWAIIAN WRISTS

This is a great movement, and once you get into the rhythm of it, you'll feel like a Hawaiian luau dancer. It becomes very flowing and you can almost hear the waves lapping in the distance.

Begin with your hands in front of your heart, and begin to rotate your wrists in soft, gentle circles. Reverse directions when you feel like it.

OPTION: As your wrists rotate away from your heart, allow them to swoop out into the distance a bit, even bringing your arms into the action.

OPTION: If your wrists feel supple and flexible, you can deepen this stretch by having your hands lightly touching as you circle your wrists. First the palms are touching, then they will roll so the backs of your hands touch, then the sides of your hands, then back to the palms and so on. Let your hands spiral out from the fulcrum point of your wrists.

This can be a deep stretch for the wrists, so absolutely do not give more than 70%. If only the tips of your fingertips can remain in contact, instead of your hands, that is excellent. Stay there and enjoy making that move as graceful as possible.

*

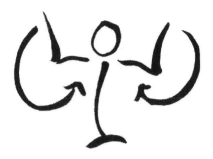

SPIRAL – ELBOWS

This is a great go-to yoga move that creates a light breeze on your face, and has a fun, swooping rhythm to it.

Begin with your arms stretched at your sides, parallel to the ground. Then point your hands upwards, while your shoulder and upper arms remain parallel to the ground. Then swoop your hands inwards toward the heart so the fingertips are facing each other. Then drop your hands down and continue circling.

Let your momentum carry this one, and remember to keep your shoulders and upper arms still and parallel to the ground, so your forearms rotate around your elbow joint. Keep your shoulders nice and relaxed.

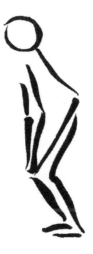

SPIRAL – KNEES

This is a nice, gentle circling motion that warms up your knee joints. It's a great warm-up before a hike or walk. It's also an excellent way to loosen up after a long time seated.

From a standing position, place your hands on your knees, bending the knees slightly. Then rotate in circles. First one way, then the other.

*

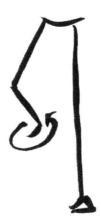

SPIRAL – ANKLES

Ankle circles can be done from a standing or seated position. They follow the same instructions as the infinity ankle rolls.

Lounging comfortably on your sofa or seated at your desk, simply lift your foot up and turn your ankle in gentle circles.

Keeping the ankle supple has great advantages, since your entire body weight depends upon the health and well-being of this often neglected joint.

If standing, you can keep one toe on the ground for balance while softly rotating your ankle. Or bring your knee up high enough that you get in a good balancing pose while spiraling your ankle in circles. Do this in a safe location in case you tip over.

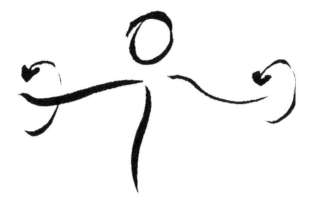

SPIRAL – WRISTS AND FOREARMS

With arms stretched out to the side, softly spiral your wrists in circles, keeping your arms and shoulders locked in position. Rotate in both directions.

OPTION: Keep your wrists locked into position, and move the length of your entire arms in circles.

This move generates from the shoulder sockets and you'll notice a nice stretch along the underside of your arm and elbow area.

Do this movement with your palms facing down, then up. The stretch when the palms are facing up is much more pronounced.

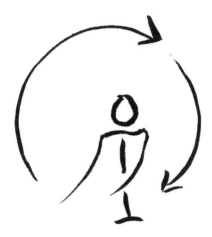

SPIRAL – PARALLEL ARM CIRCLES

This move definitely includes cardio, and you'll notice your heart rate increase after just a couple of circles.

Begin with both arms stretched out to the right. Then move them in tandem up above your head, over to your left, down and back to the right, continuing in large circles.

After eight repetitions, or whatever time frame suits you, change direction.

This is a vigorous move that really gets the blood flowing and the oxygen circulating in your entire upper body, bringing increased energy and vitality.

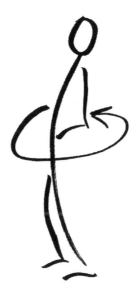

SPIRAL – HIP CIRCLES

This is a classic yoga move, great for loosening the hip area.

With hands on hips, knees slightly bent, simply rotate your hip girdle in large, luxurious circles. If you're in public, perhaps waiting in a line, practice a subtle, almost invisible version.

Both versions will improve circulation and release lower back tension. A great stretching movement to use after a long time seated.

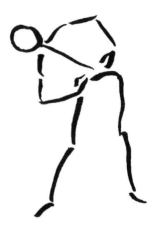

SPIRAL – TRUNK CIRCLES

While hip circles open the hips, this upper body circle targets the waist. It also massages the internal organs, aids digestion and relaxes the back muscles.

The key in this movement is to keep the lower body stable and to let the upper body rotate. Change directions halfway through.

*

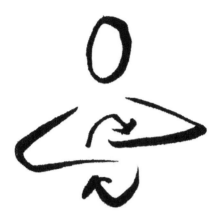

SPIRAL – FOREARM SPIRALS

This is a pleasant move that can be slow and relaxing or quick and stimulating. It's a contained movement, which makes it perfect for practicing in small spaces, such as at your desk or in your car.

Begin with your arms out in front of you, your hands meeting your opposite elbows as though you're leaning on a high counter with your arms loosely crossed. But don't let your forearms touch each other. Instead, allow them to circle around each other like an eggbeater on its side.

TIP: The upper arms remain fairly still. The hands can be held in loose fists or with the palms flat. The shoulders are relaxed.

TAYLORE DANIEL

7

Tapping

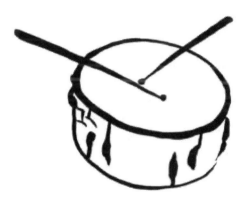

TAYLORE DANIEL

*

F.I.R.S.T.

T IS FOR TAPPING

Tapping is a relaxing yet powerful and effective activity that energizes the body, stimulates the organs, flushes out toxins, increases circulation, rejuvenates the skin, and releases stress, both physical and emotional.

Best of all, it can be practiced any time and any place, whether you're shopping, watching a movie, walking or reading a book.

You can tap your body using a loose fist, an open palm, or even with your fingertips. In fact, it's best to use only the fingertips around joints such as the elbows and knees.

Tap any part of your body randomly.

You may be surprised at just how much tension you're holding in a given area and will be able to sense the tight muscles beneath your skin when you begin tapping them.

TAPPING – LIMBS

Try tapping while stopped at traffic lights, sitting on an airplane, or at work behind your desk. Tapping up and down the tops and sides of your leg muscles feels great, as does tapping up and down your arms from above your elbow to your shoulder. Tapping your chest and stomach area is also a treat.

For a more structured tapping session, begin at the top of your shoulder, tapping with your loose fist or open palm all the way down your outer arms to your hand, then up your inside arm toward your shoulder. Do both arms.

Next, follow this same pattern down the outside of your legs and up the inside. Then tap the fronts of your legs down to your feet, and up the back of your legs.

Again, use only the fingertips around the knees and elbows. There are a number of acupressure points around these joints, so they are great areas to give more focused attention if you have the time.

TAPPING – TRUNK & HEAD

Using a loose fist, open palm or even the back of your hand, tap your lower and mid-back area. This increases circulation to the kidneys and adrenal glands, relaxes the lower back and balances the central nervous system.

Bring your hands around to your belly, still tapping. Tapping the abdomen stimulates digestion. Then continue tapping up to your chest and sternum area. This brings energy to the lungs, heart and thymus gland, which is rejuvenated by the stimulation.

Coming up to your neck, begin to lighten the tapping by using your fingertips. This relieves neck tension.

Using your fingertips to tap your scalp has the added bonus of giving the reflexology points on the end of each fingertip some attention.

TAPPING – FEET

There are more acupressure and reflexology points on your feet than anywhere else on your body, so the benefits of tapping the bottoms of your feet are manifold. Use a light fist to tap away to your heart's content.

TAPPING – FINGERS

As mentioned above, there are reflexology points on the tip of each finger. These can be tapped by pressing the thumb against each finger in turn.

The tap can be like a quick pat or a pressing together of each fingertip with the thumb. Each tap or press activates and stimulates a different part of the body. This practice is a powerhouse that can help release both physical and emotional blockages and stress throughout the body.

OPTION: Do this series of taps while walking, coordinating each step with one finger tap against the thumb.

OPTION: Add to the previous option by coordinating your breathing with the tapping of your fingers and your footsteps. Inhale to the count of four, as you take four steps and press your thumbs to each of your four fingers.

Then exhale to the count of four steps, while synchronizing four more taps of your thumbs to your fingers.

You can practice increasing your inhalations and exhalations to a count of eight steps each if this is comfortable.

Synchronizing breathing to your steps can be done for a couple of minutes here and there during a walk. It doesn't have to be for a marathon.

The specific benefits of synchronized walking/breathing/tapping include enhanced brain function and mood regulation.

Inhaling for eight and exhaling for four also increases energy. Doing the opposite, inhaling for four and exhaling to the count of eight, increases relaxation. Quite simply, exhaling brings relaxation, and inhaling brings energy.

Synchronizing your breathing to any movement also has the effect of bringing your nervous system into balance and harmony. Powerful stuff.

8

Conclusion

WAYS TO USE THIS GUIDE

The whole premise behind *The Lazy Woman's Guide to Yoga* is that you can sneak some marvelous yoga moves into your day—with no mats, special clothing or floor work involved.

Whether you're a person who feels too busy for yoga, a couch potato who has a hard time getting motivated, or a techie-driven individual who can't break away from the screen, this guide is meant to give you some fun, effortless, convenient options to add more oomph into your life.

It can be done anytime, anywhere, with complete randomness and great results.

Or if you'd like to put what you've learned from *The Lazy Woman's Guide to Yoga* into your life in a more structured way, there's a couple of neat options.

OPTION: Practice one style of movement per weekday. There are five styles in total—F.I.R.S.T.—which can be matched to the days of the week. For instance, Monday for Flying, Tuesday for Infinity, Wednesday for Rock, Thursday for Spiral and Friday for Tapping, leaving the weekend to mix and match.

An advantage of this structure is that it gives each day an extra little reminder of one category of moves. At the end of the week, you'll find you have a deeper relationship with each of the styles in F.I.R.S.T.

OPTION: Run through eight repetitions (or eight seconds) from each letter in quick succession. This can take as little as 60 seconds and is surprisingly energizing.

For instance, eight repetitions of Flying (arms up and down), eight repetitions of Infinity (maybe wrists), eight seconds of Rock (balancing on one leg or a plank), eight seconds of Spirals (perhaps eyes), eight seconds of Tapping (arms or legs).

Or for a longer blast of yoga, add more repetitions, or do three to ten minutes from each letter of F.I.R.S.T.

Personally, I love filling in the wait times that pop up

throughout the day with mini-yoga breaks, such as when my computer is booting up, the elevator is rising, the traffic light is on red... all those moments that I'd otherwise be passively waiting.

Slipping yoga between my daily activities acts as a reset button, reminding me how much I love moving my body while otherwise living my life effortlessly... even lazily.

Quite simply: F.I.R.S.T. things first. Flying. Infinity. Rock. Spiral. Tapping.

*

FLYING

INFINITY

ROCK

SPIRAL

TAPPING

Acknowledgements

With sincere appreciation for the support and encouragement of wonderful friends and family, and for the fabulous yoga community in Vancouver.

A special thanks to my partner. He makes it all possible. He makes it all meaningful. He makes it all worthwhile.

About the Author

Taylore Daniel is a yoga teacher, public speaker and travel writer who has traveled through thirty countries, using yoga to stay healthy and energized on the road.

To book a speaking engagement or workshop with Taylore, or to share your comments and stories, please contact her at www.tayloredaniel.com

OTHER BOOKS BY TAYLORE DANIEL

"The Lazy Man's Guide to Yoga"

50366204R00060

Made in the USA
San Bernardino, CA
21 June 2017